Contents

Introduction

CBD, generally alluded to as cannabidiol, can be drawn out from the hemp or cannabis plants. A huge number of research thinks about performed in the course of the most recent couple of years are uncovering that CBD may have a vast scope of recuperating points of interest, albeit more research is required.

It's difficult to switch on the news nowadays without hearing reports of cannabis and hemp being sanctioned far and wide - and with incredible reason: these 2 plants have been essential to mankind as prescriptions, nourishment, fuel, fiber and more for incalculable years. They're especially sheltered, develop very and consummately in numerous atmospheres, and have an uncommon rundown of valuable uses. It's as though Mother Nature created them just for us.

Furthermore, as a general rule, that is not an amazingly fantastical idea. The body really contains extraordinary receptors all through the nerve framework that are explicitly activated by substances found basically in the cannabis and hemp plants. Like, for example, CBD (Cannabidiol), a fringe wonderful aggravate that is by and by being vigorously researched far and wide and is uncovering promising signs as a potential treatment for some significant ailments in both creature and human models, notwithstanding an all out wellbeing protectant and sponsor.

Despite the fact that it's too soon to make any authoritative wellbeing claims with respect to precisely what CBD can or can't do, the examination around the substance is utilizing a look into potential mending utilizes, some of which we'll investigate beneath, and episodic reports from huge quantities of individuals around the globe program that without a doubt there is something one of a kind about CBD oil. Inning understanding with Nora Volkow, the chief of the National Institute on Drug Abuse, "Thorough logical examinations are as yet expected to assess the therapeutic capability of CBD for explicit conditions. All things considered, pre-clinical research (comprising of both cell culture and creature plans) has really uncovered CBD to have a progression of effects that might be remedially useful, including against seizure, cancer prevention agent, neuroprotective, mitigating, pain relieving, hostile to tumor, against insane, and against nervousness properties."

Evidently Cannabidiol has a great deal taking the plunge. The street ahead will incorporate twofold visually impaired human clinical preliminaries to check or deny these early discoveries that certainly show up amazingly engaging. Nonetheless, meanwhile, that has not halted wellbeing searchers worldwide from taking in CBD with the expectation that they may exploit its alleged impacts - and various are revealing positive encounters in accordance with precisely what the analysts are finding.

THE HISTORY:

For over 10,000 years, the Cannabis / Hemp plant has provided humankind with food, fiber, inebriation and medicine. We know this because of plants found in ancient areas of the Middle East and Asia in clay jars dated over 10,000 years old.

Cannabinoids, the medicinally active substances produced within the Hemp plant, influence and interact with specific receptors of the human body. There are receptors in the body and brain which are affected differently. There are many varieties of cannabis which express different chemistries that affect the body and mind differently and provide unique healing properties as well. Some have high THC (psychoactive abilities) and low CBD (non-psychoactive) and vice versa. CBD has been proven to be effective with little to no high. CBD is just the acronym for Cannabidiol one of 119 Cannabinoids found in Hemp.

Asian traditions alone document Cannabis as an important herbal medicine over 4,700 years ago. History suggests it was first used as a spice well before it was heated, smoked and liquefied as a type of butter. Hemp and Cannabis were used extensively in the United States from approximately 1830 as anti-inflammatories and other beneficial medicines. Further it was used to help with pain well before the chemicals of the pharmaceutical industry took over to block signals to the brain artificially. J.R Reynolds the personal physician to Queen Victoria wrote in his respected medical journal that "In almost all painful maladies,

I have found Indian Hemp by far the most useful of drugs". In 1925 the League of Nations ratified the International Opium Convention, which included language banning Cannabis and its derivatives except for medical and scientific use. Years later by

1938 it was banned in all 48 states and the powers that "were" pushed the perception for decades as a dangerous narcotic through fear-mongering and false data forcing it underground and into then into cartels.

In the early 1900's farmers were given "certificate of value" for their Hemp grown. It was a common unit for farming textiles, paper, rope clothing, building materials and more. Eventually in the late 1960's through scientific research in Jerusalem the powerful psychoactive ingredient was uncovered in the Cannabis plant and was called delta-9-tetrahydrocannabinoid (THC). Hemp, unlike Cannabis has very low amounts of "naturally occurring" THC in the plant and is therefore more recognized as medicinal. Hemp is also an amazingly unique plant with abilities to be useful, robust and flexible and was used for clothing, sails for ships, paper and an innumerable other uses all over the world in the 1800's. Hemp seed oils were also used for hundreds of medicinal purposes.

Hemp is a "remarkable" plant that is an efficient Bio-Remediator which means that when planted will actually remove toxins from the soil around it. Hemp uses significantly less water than other crops. Additionally, it grows with minimal to no fertilizer, pesticides and herbicides. Glyphosate is the poison that is used as a pesticide (Monsanto Corp) in crops and has been linked to Autism,

Alzheimer's and many other conditions in the human brain.

Since research on the human genome has proven that 90% of all diseases come from environmental factors – a clean environment can improve health & wellness for all of us. Hemp and Cannabis are in the

same plant family, but very different plants. Think of a Tiger and a Panther, both cats but "very" different.

CANNABIDIOL

CBD is one of over 80 compounds found in the Hemp plant that belong to a class of molecules called Cannabinoids. Of these compounds, CBD and THC are usually present in the highest concentrations, and are therefore the most recognized and studied. Since 1980 more research has been done and findings have been expanding on the wide range of benefits. To this end, much data was hidden from mainstream as during the 80's and 90's the Pharmaceutical industry was flourishing creating jobs and economic profits. Only until the first few states in the US voted to legalize medical Cannabis were the results and studies eventually published and understood.

CBD and THC levels tend to vary among different plants and are just part of these remarkable chemical ecologies which contain dozens of medicinally active substances.

This variation in potency and constituency along with complex chemical interactions, further combined with the way the human body metabolizes them, make it very difficult to determine a clear scale of dosage. The health benefits of Cannabidiol are well established with more information coming each day.

All mammals have an "endo-cannabinoid system" that exists naturally in the body and works in concert with the immune system to regulate and fight infections. This ECS (Endo-Cannabinoid System) is a group of endogenous cannabinoid receptors located in the bran and throughout the central and peripheral nervous systems, consisting of neuromodulatory lipids and their receptors. CBD specifically interacts with the CB1 and CB2 receptors that send signals to wake up and strengthen the immune system naturally. This is because our endocannabinoid system is intricately linked to our nervous system and immune system, as well as our brain and digestive system via the Vegus nerve. Quality CBD is an effective form of alternative natural treatment to many ailments and illnesses of various types. While these statements have not been reviewed or confirmed by the FDA, there is much in the US that has been proven to be beneficial with no confirmation by the FDA. Additionally, there are in fact many substances that have been proven to be toxic and dangerous to the human body and have been approved by the FDA, so do your own research and get educated on both.

Not only does CBD stimulate the immune system, but Cannabidiol (CBD) works to help counteract the psychoactive properties of THC and its brain/body altering effects. In its raw form it is an oily substance that is extracted from seeds, leaves and stock of the Hemp plant. CBD is gaining much awareness and word of mouth is spreading from the people who have turned to

CBD for ailments instead of prescription meds and are seeing significant results.

For this reason it is vital to be sure you are buying CBD from a reputable source since many low-grade CBD formulas are being sold for high profits. These lower grade CBD formulas contain fillers including Progesterone and are not as beneficial as pure Hemp CBD. Recently I had a client come into the store with a 60mil bottle of 3,000mg CBD and said she took two full droppers with no effect. Two full droppers of 3,000mg CBD would equate to 100mg of CBD. I had the bottle tested and it came back at 4.066mg per mil meaning there was less than 300mg in the entire bottle.

We have also had a lot of people buying online with the same result. Buyer beware and never underestimate the power of greed in people.

The CBD molecule is very different tha n the THC molecule and operates within the body in a different way.

Major Benefits of CBD

Multiple Sclerosis and other conditions that cause seizures have been treated with CBD with positive results. Some of the other maladies are

Acne

Pain

Diabetes

Insomnia

Anxiety

Depression

Migraines

Asthma

Scar tissue

Crohn's Disease

Schizophrenia

Alzheimer's

Parkinson's

Nausea

Neuropathy

PTSD

Skin Conditions

Chronic Fatigue Syndrome

Auto Immune Disorders

Attention Deficit Disorder Hyperactivity

Fibromyalgia

Colitis

Cancer.

CBD and FAAH

Unlike psychoactive THC, CBD has little binding affinity to either the CB1 or CB2 cannabinoid receptors. Instead, CBD indirectly stimulates endogenous cannabinoid signaling by suppressing the enzyme fatty acid amide hydroxylase (FAAH)—the enzyme that breaks down anandamide, the first endocannabinoid discovered in the mammalian brain in 1992.

Whereas the cannabinoid molecules found in cannabis are considered "exogenous ligands" to the cannabinoid (CB) receptor family, anandamide is an "endogenous" cannabinoid ligand—meaning it binds to one or more cannabinoid receptors and is found naturally inside the mammalian brain and body. Anandamide favors the CB1 receptor, which is concentrated in the brain and central nervous system. Because FAAH is involved in the metabolic breakdown of anandamide, less FAAH means more anandamide remains present in the body for a longer duration. More anandamide means greater CB1 activation.

CBD enhances endocannabinoid tone by suppressing FAAH. By inhibiting the enzyme that metabolizes and degrades anandamide, CBD enhances the body's innate protective endocannabinoid response. At the same time, CBD opposes the action of THC at the CB1 receptor site, thereby muting the psychoactive effects of THC. CBD also stimulates the release of 2-AG, another endocannabinoid that activates both CB1 and CB2 receptor.

CB2 receptors are predominant in the peripheral nervous system and the immune system. CBD has been shown to directly interact with other "G-protein-coupled" receptors and ion channels to confer a therapeutic effect. CBD, for example, binds to the TRPV-1 receptor, which is known to mediate pain perception, inflammation and body temperature.

The Serotonin Receptor

Jose Alexandre Crippa and his colleagues at the University of San Paulo in Brazil and at the King's College in London have conducted pioneering research into CBD and the neural correlates of anxiety. At high concentrations, CBD directly activates the 5-HT1A (hydroxytryptamine) serotonin receptor, thereby conferring an anti-depressant effect. This receptor is implicated in a range of biological and neurological processes, including (but not limited to) anxiety, addiction, appetite, sleep, pain perception, nausea and vomiting. This is why we have been so successful helping people wean off depression medications with CBD.

NEURO-INNFLAMMATION EPIDEMIC

Micro-glia is an immune cell in the brain which is attacked by Astrocytes that get into the brain from environmental sources and causes neuro-inflammation. When you take CBD, you are assisting your body's natural ability to pool up or increase the production of Anandamide as well as the family of Glutathion. This increase in Glutathion influences 3 things

1. Antioxidants

2. Detoxification

3. Protein repair

Additionally CBD helps to turn down Gene's that are pro-inflammatory like EMF stress or Peroxy Nitrates and other VOC's like air pollution.

The best education you can get about Phospholipids is Bruce Lipton's work. Bruce Lipton is a Cellular biologist who proved that the cell does not die when you remove the nucleus. Epigenetic's and Membranes are fascinating to study...after all; it's how your body works.

The intelligence or Brain within the cell is not in the nucleus. This was believed to be the case for decades. Bruce proved otherwise. The Nucleus is just the vault or library that holds or stores all the "potential" that your genes offer. But it's the membrane that "reads" the environment. This is our energy, which includes our thoughts, both subconscious and conscious, nutrients and any toxins that may be present in our system. Remember we are both chemical and electrical beings. So the membrane decides what is needed based on the condition. If we DO NOT have the resources within our body to stop this aberrant condition, it goes on. With CBD, we are simply providing another natural phyto-nutrient to the mix that will allow these membranes to have the resources needed to stop pain, anxiety or help heal that particular condition. It is vital to feed our cells the stuff that they need to function. We need healthy phospholipids. When cells are not fed right they become damaged, and they cannot function optimally. This is why CBD doesn't work for some people at low doses. It will work, you just have damaged cells and need more dose. A better diet helps CBD work better at low doses.

Cells are made up of Organelles. All of the Organelles are made up of Membranes. Membranes function with electrical and chemical balance. We have videos on our You Tube page about how to increase your electrical charge. Energy is used throughout the entire body to drive enzymatic reaction. Mitochondria are the energy factories of the cells. This energy-rich molecule is called ATP or Adenosine triphosphate. ATP is produced in the mitochondria using energy stored in food.

This is called Electron Transport Chain ETC. Damaged cells cannot operate properly to regulate homeostasis.

IS IT LEGAL?

You will hear or read that CBD is illegal in the United States, but this statement is currently untrue depending on the potency and other factors. Some CBD has high level of tetrahydrocannabinoid (THC) which does make it illegal as a Schedule I drug in the United States.

There is one important statute to "understand". As long as there is less than .3% THC in the pharmaceutical grade CBD, then it falls under the exemption of Drug Enforcement Admin 357 F.3d 1012 (9th cir. 2004) CSA definition of marijuana but recently the government has become more involved with regard to Hemp-based CBD and unfortunately for all of us may soon be taken from us over the counter. Stay involved and help us keep this low cost natural medication legal for all of us.

The Legal "Break Down"

Marijuana is currently listed as a Schedule I narcotic under the federal Controlled Substances Act, meaning the federal government believes it to be a dangerous drug with no recognized medical benefit. Consequently, any CBD derived from marijuana violates the federal Controlled Substances Act, and the Drug Enforcement Administration has already stated that it believes CBD to be a marijuana derivative and, therefore, a Schedule I drug.

Hemp, on the other hand, is more complicated. The DEA defines hemp as the parts of the cannabis plant excluded from the Controlled Substances Act, namely the mature stalks and seeds. To legally grow cannabis in the U.S. — hemp or not — you must possess a permit from the DEA. Consequently, cultivating hemp without a permit remains a federal crime. The only exception is the 2014 federal Farm Bill, which defines "industrial hemp" as cannabis that contains less than 0.3 percent THC by weight, and which allows state departments of agriculture, universities, and colleges to cultivate industrial hemp for educational and research purposes without a DEA permit. Despite the prohibition on hemp cultivation without a DEA-issued permit, it is not a violation of the federal Controlled Substances Act to purchase, sell, and possess processed hemp products.

In the 2005 case of Hemp Industries Association v. Drug Enforcement Administration, the Ninth Circuit held that the DEA had gone beyond its mandate in attempting to regulate all products containing any amount of THC because "Congress did not regulate non-psychoactive hemp in Schedule I." The Ninth Circuit further held that "the DEA's action is not a mere classification of its THC regulations; it improperly renders naturally-occurring non-psychoactive hemp illegal for the first time."

The court concluded that Congressional intent was, "unambiguous... with regard to the regulation of non-psychoactive hemp," and ruled that the DEA "cannot regulate naturally-occurring THC not contained within or derived from marijuana — i.e., non-psychoactive hemp products-because non-psychoactive hemp is not included in Schedule I."

Because of the DEA's general prohibition on any cannabis cultivation, most hemp products we see in the U.S. are imported from overseas. And, as a result of the Hemp Industries Association case, companies and individuals may freely sell CBD derived from processed hemp (not from marijuana), imported from outside the U.S. Notably, the Food and Drug Administration (FDA) has also inserted itself into the CBD market. Generally, when a company makes a medical claim about a product, that product is classified as a drug. Under the Federal Food, Drug and Cosmetic Act (FDAC), new drugs are not allowed to enter the market without first being FDA-tested (unless they meet the definition of a dietary supplement). When these types of medical claims are made without the requisite testing, the FDA takes action under the FDAC.

The FDA does not consider CBD to be a dietary supplement; it considers CBD to be a new drug. As a result, earlier this year, the FDA issued warning letters to companies making specific medical claims about their CBD products. The

FDA accused these companies of making unfounded medical and therapeutic claims about their CBD products by, for instance, stating that CBD is effective for treating certain kinds of cancer even though many people were seeing significant benefits. The FDA gave these companies 15 days to demonstrate how they were curing their violations or face legal action by the FDA.

Anyone undertaking to sell hemp-derived CBD should make clear to regulators and to its customers that its products come from imported or domestic hemp and not from marijuana. Moreover, anyone selling or making hemp-derived CBD should also avoid making any specific medical claims about those products. At this point it's up to the people to try it and form their own conclusions.

Logic dictates (exempt from the FDA) if people were not seeing results, the popularity would not be at its current level. How can the FDA ignore a Parkinson's patient that takes CBD and stops shaking in 2 minutes? Simple, it costs Big Pharma billions!

It is IMPORTANT that everyone understand how the FDA came to be and what they actually do. This link to a short documentary will help you understand that most government agencies including the American Medical Association do not exist to just "help" consumers. They control the entire healthcare industry including Pharma which is financial "profit" based. Everyone should spend 14 minutes learning a few things about these organizations.

The FDA pays Big Pharma to fast track drugs to market.

DOSING

What is the proper amount of CBD to ingest? There is no specific amount for each person. Each person is unique, like a snowflake. Start with a specific dose and monitor for 3 – 5 days. Most people start with 5 to 10 Mg's per day. CBD does build up in your system to get the full effect, like a multi vitamin. Start between 5 to 20mg per day and monitor. If you require more, you can slowly increase the dose. Be aware of yourself and your symptoms and always monitor your body. It is not unlike a workout routine that you monitor and write down your reps and sets so you can adjust as needed based on how your body responds. Obviously it goes without saying that any "dis" ease in the body means something is not working optimally.

You must be serious about "healing yourself" and never underestimate the power of your will.

Your intention and your will play a role in your health at all times and stress is a killer.

CBD is a compound that works at the cellular level so it doesn't mask symptoms like pharmaceutical drugs. There are many things you can do to heal such as increase raw food diet, increase your protein intake and meditation. Add pure Ascorbic Acid and Baking Soda to your daily routine, all which help put your body in a "state" to heal optimally. When toxins and negative energy like drama and stress are removed, the body can do what is was divinely inspired to do and heal.

High quality CBD is not cheap so only use what your body needs. The higher the milligram, the more it will cost.

A review published in Current Drug Safety concluded that CBD "does not interfere with several psychomotor and psychological functions." The authors add that several studies suggest that CBD is "well tolerated and safe" even at very high doses.

This video is a short Beginners Guide to Hemp-based CBD Oils, Capsules, and Concentrates.

https://www.youtube.com/watch?v=8tJW5 W6gaxo&t=30s

HOW TO INGEST?

There are many ways you can ingest CBD. You may utilize CBD in edible form such as gummies, capsules, or candies. We don't recommend gummies/candies as they have sugar and other additives which is part of the problem with human health. We don't need more preservatives and sugar in our bodies. There is a crumble, which is a waxy solid that requires heating to liquefy for consumption and requires a ceramic vaporizer to inhale. The delivery when inhaled is much faster than when consumed through the digestive tract. See Video Link below. There are also capsules, creams and sprays. Another type of CBD is concentrate which is a more "raw" form of CBD and is a powder or otherwise referred to as an isolate. This isolate can be eaten or liquefied or vaped.

There are liquid forms of CBD (the most popular) which are formulated with coconut

oil or vegetable glycerin and are referred to as intra oral or "sublingual" and placed under the tongue before swallowing.

Yes you may give small doses of CBD to your pets to help them remain healthy. CBD can be used in all mammals for health. Pet treats are also a gimmick as they also have preservatives. Just use the same pure CBD you take on your pet in a much lower dose. If you choose to vape CBD, there are many choices including pre-packaged cartridges.

Part of being a healthy person is to always be utilizing "all" your sensory abilities. Taste, smell, touch, and hearing are important faculties. Classical music and Jazz are proven to be healing at a cellular level.

Heavy metal and Rapp music are not healing and place the body in an "alert" fight or flight state increasing adrenaline and are not relaxing to the body and mind.

CB1 AND CB2 RECEPTORS

There are receptors in the body and brain which are stimulated differently depending on how you choose to absorb the CBD. The two primary subtypes of CBD receptors are CB1 and CB2. These receptors are distributed throughout the central, peripheral, nervous and immune system and are present in various tissues including the brain, gastrointestinal system, reproductive and urinary tracts, spleen, endocrine system, heart and circulatory system. Recently researchers have uncovered new evidence that points to at least three other Cannabinoid receptors throughout the body.

Following the discovery of these cannabinoid receptors, the hunt was on to find the substances produced in the human body that were binding to them. This led to the discovery of the first endocannabinoids, "anandamide and 2-AG, in the early 1900's.

So far to date five endocannabinoids have been isolated. All of them are derivatives of the polyunsaturated fatty acids, closely related to the very popular Omega-3 fatty acids. These Omega-3 fatty acids are the same people often purchase at health food stores for vitamin supplements. Since they are fats, endocannabinoids are not water-soluble and therefore have trouble moving quickly throughout the body. For this reason they are designed to work locally. One of these important local activities occurs when endocannabinoids serve as the primary messenger across synapsis (the gaps between nerve cells). They signal neurons to communicate with each other through the release of neurotransmitters in the brain. It has become clear in recent years that the role of endocannabinoids in the synaptic function is both more important and far more complex than previously thought. Endocannabinoids modulate the flow of neurotransmitters,

running smoothly. Our cannabinoids are produced on demand and then taken up into the cells and rapidly metabolized. Our cannabinoids appear to be profoundly connected with the concept of homeostasis which is defined as "maintaining physiological stability". It basically helps redress specific imbalances presented by disease or by injury. It is also believed that the endocannabinoid levels may be responsible for the baseline of pain throughout the body. This is why CBD medicines are helpful in treating conditions such as Fibromyalgia (a condition marked by muscular pain).

This could also mean that the constant release of the body's own endocannabinoids have a "tonic" effect on muscle tightness in Multiple Sclerosis, neuropathic pain, inflammation and even appetite. Thus the "value" of the endocannabinoid system throughout the body is very significant in general overall well-being.

The CB1 receptor is expressed throughout the brain, where it works in concert with the endocannabinoid system to form a "circuit breaker" which modulates the release of neurotransmitters. The list of brain functions that are affected by this system is enormous and too large for this book. Just a few are here: Movement, cognition, emotions, decision making, learning, memory, regulation of body movement and functions, anxiety, fear, stress, pain, and more.

One brain region which does not have any CB1 receptors is the brain stem, responsible for respiration and circulation. This is why cannabis in high doses are not fatal. To date there has never been one documented case of a cannabis related death from over dose. Compare that to Prescription drugs. It is the "activation" of the CB1 receptor that is
responsible for the psychoactive effects of cannabis. The CB2 receptor does not have this effect. The CB2 receptors are primarily found in the blood cells, Tonsils and the Spleen. From these sites CB2 receptors control the release of cytokines or immunoregulatory proteins linked to inflammation and general immune functions. This is why quality Protein is important to the human body as it provides the building blocks of your cells and immune system. This is a massive book on its own.

People consume far too little "quality" protein and far too much Alcohol in this country.

The healthcare system will "never" be balanced until people begin to take more responsibility for their own health and stop relying on pills.

CBD AND DRUG TESTING

A routine urine drug screen for marijuana use consists of an immunoassay with antibodies that are made to detect it, and its main metabolite, 11-nor-delta9-caboxy-THC (THC-COOH). The cutoff level for a positive urine screen in the immunoassay at 50 ng/mL. When the immunoassay screen is positive at the > 50 ng/mL level, a confirmatory GC/MS The Gas Chromatography/Mass Spectrometry test is performed to verify the positive urine screen. The confirmatory GC/MS has a cutoff level of 15 ng/mL and is specific only to the 11-nor-THCCOOH metabolite. Fortunately, the urine drug screen for THC-COOH is known to have very little cross-reactivity to other cannabinoids that are not psychoactive, such as CBD (cannabidiol), CBG (cannabigerol), CBN (cannabinol).

Individuals using unusually large doses of a cannabinoid-rich hemp oil product (above 1000-2000 mg of hemp oil daily) could theoretically test positive during the initial urinary screen. The urine screen in these cases would likely represent a "false positive" due to other non-THC metabolites or compounds, which may cross-react with the immunoassay. Keep in mind that most of the high-quality, reliable CBD-rich hemp oil products contain much less THC than marijuana. Hemp contains anywhere from 1/10th to 1/300th of the THC concentration found in marijuana. An individual consuming 1000-2000 mg per day of hemp oil would thus consume about 3-6 mg of THC-A. THC-A is the compound found in Cannabis prior to being decarboxylated (heated to release the psychoactive affects) Raw Cannabis does not get you high.

Exceedingly high dose may result in detection of positive urine screen in up to 11% to 23% of assays.

Note: Most research suggests that for infrequent or 'non-daily' users of cannabis,

a typical high-dose marijuana cigarette (containing about 40mg to 50mg of THC) would result in a positive THC metabolite screen for up to two days at this cutoff level.

This depends on many factors including:

1. How much & how often cannabis is used

2. The metabolism of each individual

3. The route of administration

4. Other factors such as medications used, liver or kidney disease.

5. Body type, H2O, various organic liquid antioxidant consumption.

Data based on SAMHSA standards. If you have any concern about testing positive for THC when using CBD please seek advice from your health care professional.

New data suggest that it may be possible for CBD to convert to THC in the stomach. Here are the details on this new finding as of November 2017.

Through much research it appears that stomach acid can "potentially" convert CBD to THC at low levels. This has implications for people who consume CBD and for those who have to take or receive random drug tests. There seems to be one caveat worth noting regarding this finding. Full spectrum Hemp oils high in CBD seem to be the primary culprit since they contain all the plant material including CBD, CBG and CBN as well and trace amounts of other cannabinoids. This data could have repercussions for a small segment of people consuming CBD.

Remember, this will not occur using a topical method of delivery since there would be no exposure to stomach acids with a topical or even inhaling it.

"Gastric fluid enzymes can convert CBD into the psychoactive components D9-THC and D8-THC, which suggests that the oral route of administration may increase the potential for positive immune essay or even a false positive which is common.

First, if you ask a synthetic organic chemist if it was possible to convert CBD to THC under highly acidic conditions they would say "yes, but the yields are low". Second, while the stomach is acidic (pH 2) almost Hydrochloric Acid the rest of the GI is weakly acidic to neutral (pH 5.7 -7.4), which disfavors the conversion (it can still happen but only very slowly).

Finally, some enzymes can also do this conversion independent of pH. So, do these enzymes exist in the GI system? Yes for some and no for others. Gastric enzymes is a massive topic since each person is 100% unique, and the types and amounts of foods they consume are rarely exactly the same... therefore this requires a lot more study.

The answer at least temporarily maybe to consume only 100% pure CBD from the Isolate and not the full Spectrum. This may help mitigate the "potential" for your body to have any conversion in the stomach per your unique gastric juices.

UNDERSTANDING TERPENES

Terpenoids, otherwise known as terpenes, are a category of phytochemicals produced by many plants including hemp that are believed to possess a wide range of therapeutic benefits. Terpenes are natural chemicals found in every plant on Earth. Plants evolved with unique chemical profiles for protection and humans evolved to use plants for homeostasis, therapy and enjoyment. Although much is known about terpenes and their medical and recreational use (aromatherapies) even more is unknown about the chemical synergies that produce the entourage effect. The cannabis plant contains over 200 known terpenes to date.

These terpenes act synergistically with the cannabinoids, like CBD and also THC, to create the therapeutic effects. These flavor profiles are created by the biochemical secreted in the trichome's of cannabis along with cannabinoids found in the Hemp Plant.

Hemp contains over 200 terpenes, some of which are in the therapeutically significant range of over 0.05%, though the terpenes reaching this concentration vary by strain. One of these terpenes is the aptly named terpinolene. Terpinolene is also found in apple, cumin, lilac and tea tree, and has a smoky or woody scent. It is the terpenes, not the cannabinoids that are responsible for the aroma of hemp plants.

NON-CANNABIS CANNABINOIDS

Yes, there are other plant compounds that contain powerful Cannabinoids and we will have these new medications very soon. I'm so excited to share this new product with our many clients.

SOME FACTS TO SHARE

The National Poison Data System produces a report on various deaths. The 174-page detailed report indicated that the number of Americans killed in 2009 by vitamins, minerals, amino acids or herbal supplements was zero.

There were 300,000 deaths from "auto" wrecks. This number is rising due to mobile devices distracting people constantly.

There were at least 1.5 million Americans who got cancer and more than half died from it. That's 750,000 people dying of a preventable and curable cellular disorder. Additionally there were 375,000 deaths from heart disease and 140,000 deaths from strokes.

Alzheimer's and Dementia were the sixth leading cause of death that has a grip on over five million Americans right now and kills one in every three seniors.

More patients are dying from associated symptoms of chemotherapy and radiation than the cancer itself. Social Media, the Media and the NFL are raising awareness with pink ribbons and clothing, but it actually does nothing to "cure" cancer. There has been a massive increase in the number of people going to their doctor for Cancer screenings. Yes proactive screenings are good but few people realize that there are many doctors who make choices based on earning money for their respective departments, their board of directors, as well as their own salary to benefit their family. There have been "many" cancer cures that have never made it to the mainstream media for unknown reasons.

Google Hydrogen Peroxide Therapy for Cancer or B-17 for Cancer and see what you get. Google Hemp for skin cancer and see what you get.

There are over 2 million jobs associated with the Cancer industry and countless billions of dollars that will never cease to exist for Big Pharma. Michelin made a tire that would run over 300,000 miles but decided to not sell them. Why? Simple, lower sales revenues do not increase profits.

You must be responsible for your own health and well-being. You have obviously decided to begin your quest otherwise you would not be reading this booklet. The truth is that you need to educate yourself to the wide range of holistic sciences that exist including, CBD, Cannabis, Meditation, Hydrogen Peroxide therapies, Oxygen Healing Therapies, Baking Soda therapies and UVBI.

I would also like to share a You Tube video with you. Bruce Lipton is a world renowned cellular biologist who has proven that the way you think affects you cells. I highly recommend that you watch his lecture online for free titled "Bruce Lipton The Biology of Belief". You will be educated and amazed at how the human body works and that you have a "direct effect" on the way your cells function. This is literally life changing. With prescription medication and opiate overdoses off the charts, and over 20 million people each year being overly prescribed antibiotics it is time to begin the self-education resonance.

The Health Benefits of CBD

What The Research is Showing

So just precisely what is so incredible about CBD oil's advantages that is causing a ton intrigue and research in both the logical and therapeutic networks? To comprehend that effectively, it's critical to see how CBD functions in the psyche and body.

Neuroprotective and Antioxidant Effects

Of all CBD's archived outcomes a standout amongst its most novel and fascinating is neuroprotection, which is thought to originate from its ability to work as an incredible cell reinforcement in the cerebrum.

Neuroprotection freely alludes to the capacity of Cannabidiol- - as appeared in an assortment of creature contemplates - to a) counteract, moderate, turn around or disturb some of the methodology that outcome in the breakdown of nerve cells in the cerebrum and sensory system thought to cause numerous normal illnesses as alzheimer Parkinson's, MS, strokes and that's only the tip of the iceberg, and b) limit swelling in the mind, which is thought by various specialists to ruin cerebrum work and contribute covertly ailments like ceaseless tiredness and mind haze.

Albeit neuroprotective effects have very just been appeared creature models and cell societies, there is trust that CBD may apply comparable effects in people, however more research is required.

Hostile to Anxiety and Mood Enhancement

A standout amongst the most detectable outcomes that bunches of individuals report in the wake of taking CBD oil is a lovely and incredible decrease in pressure and tension and a noticeable lift in perspective. Bunches of clarify feeling an influx of quiet and joy washing over their bodies, which pursues CBD's accounted for results at 5-HT receptors that deal with the arrival of loads of fundamental synapses that influence pressure/tension dimensions and state of mind, especially serotonin.

One investigation of CBD separate on nervousness utilized practical attractive reverberation imaging (fMRI), which is a propelled cerebrum action mapping instrument, to think about what jumped out at the mind when people took 600mg of CBD extricate while being presented to pressure and uneasiness actuating boosts. What they found was that CBD loosened up the amygdala and cingulate cortex, 2 urgent areas of the cerebrum mainstream to oversee dread, strain levels and stress and tension, to give some examples things.

In another exploration examine, Brazilian researchers examined the consequence of CBD separate on human cortisol levels in eleven volunteers. They found that CBD diminished cortisol levels essentially more than the fake treatment which most subjects moreover detailed a soothing impact from the treatment.

In a meta-examination of CBD's effects on tension performed in Brazil, researchers found that "contemplates using creature plans of uneasiness and including sound volunteers evidently prescribe an anxiolytic-like aftereffect of CBD. Furthermore,

Cannabidiol extricate was uncovered to diminish uneasiness in patients with social tension issue."

Therefore, CBD is likewise being explored as a characteristic stimulant, hostile to insane, and a choice to SSRI meds (Prozac, and so on.).

Mitigating and Pain Reduction

Different creature considers have demonstrated that CBD has an astounding capacity to diminish explicit cell forms that bring about swelling and, accordingly, torment.

Researchers are right now completing exploration concentrates to see exactly how much this effect exchanges over to people, anyway there have really been various logical preliminaries in Europe on an item called Sativex, which is a 1:1 blend of CBD and THC.

These exploration examines found that Sativex had the capacity to bring down agony identified with focal and fringe neuropathy, rheumatoid joint inflammation, and malignant growth to changing degrees in a large portion of the examination members. It is hazy exactly the amount of an outcome Cannabidiol has on torment decline in these cases, in any case, the creature thinks about propose that CBD is likely included somewhat dependent on its perceived effects on cell forms.

In spite of the fact that the jury is still out about how powerful CBD oils and concentrates are for swelling, loads of who have been fighting with irritation related sickness like joint pain have detailed that CBD oils, concentrates and creams comprising of CBD have really helped in diminishing a couple of their signs.

Squeamishness, Diabetes, Epilepsy and others

Despite the fact that not as run of the mill, considers on creatures and a couple of, little human investigations (on account of epilepsy) moreover discovered that Cannabidiol indicates vow as a potential treatment for seizures, diabetes and queasiness, to give some examples things, albeit more research ponder is required.

Three of the 4 human investigations done using CBD as a treatment for epilepsy indicated positive results, by and by, due to make blemishes and nonattendance of meticulousness, numerous researchers are recommending that the at present promptly accessible data is deficient to reach firm determinations seeing the viability of CBD as a treatment for seizures.

Studies are at present in progress to get much better information dependent on primer engaging lead to creature preliminaries.

Psychospiritual Effects

While the psychospiritual impacts of (weed) are amazing, CBD is a later, less usually used compound, along these lines its effects and favorable circumstances in this area aren't totally seen yet. So, as referenced beforehand, many feel a stamped sedation and even sentiments of satisfaction or broad unwinding in the wake of expending top quality CBD oils and concentrates.

All things considered, CBD oil is often used by meditators to "go further, faster" as it can help with a couple of the psychological babble that much of the time surfaces amid training. Others report that the surprising, positive move in outlook that CBD oil can create is valuable in observing life from an alternate perspective that multiple occasions fits new experiences, thoughts, and conclusion about things that some time ago disturbed them.

Quality and Potency

More so than different herbs and plants, quality can be a worry with specific CBD items, so it's imperative to search out brands with a high level of security that unmistakably disclose their sourcing practices and quality principles. Search for things that are totally characteristic or possibly contain natural CBD as these are guaranteed to be without harming synthetic compounds and solvents that are frequently used in the extraction methodology of less-trustworthy organizations simply out to make a buck.

All usually offered, lawful CBD things are extricated from the hemp plant, and especially hemp oil, though items that are legitimate in certain spots however unlawful in others (contingent upon local purview) are frequently drawn out from weed (cannabis) plants and incorporate extensive and shifting dimensions of THC.

There is some proof that rates of THC increment the proficiency of CBD, in any case, it isn't required to receive the rewards of taking Cannabidiol. Research think about has uncovered unadulterated CBD removes from hemp and hemp oil, as long as the CBD is of high caliber, are likewise effective and helpful. In any case, in progressively genuine, relentless medical issues there might be extra advantages from having THC in the blend, for example, increasingly articulated uneasiness decline and therapeutic effects, inning agreement with the diverse human investigations did on the substance.

It is similarly critical to consider quality while choosing CBD things as well. Generally, the impacts of CBD are portion dependent somewhat, proposing that the more that is devoured, the more articulated its outcomes are. In that capacity, it's basic to search for increasingly focused and additionally very absorbable things for ideal impact. There are a wide assortment of Cannabidiol item potencies promptly accessible, yet an extraordinary beginning stage for most of individuals is for one measurement of the thing to be in the 2mg to 7mg assortment, with the last being on the more dominant side.

On the off chance that you realize you will in general be sensitive to characteristic items and prescriptions, start at a lower portion. On the off chance that you don't tend to feel anything or comprehend you need a more grounded item to see the benefits of CBD, don't hesitate regardless higher measurements. For some CBD hemp oil things, you can take an incomplete or twofold measurement to alter the adequacy.

CBD oil is strikingly protected and has uncovered itself to be sensibly symptom free so there's nothing to worry over except if you have a known unfavorably susceptible response to hemp or you are on some sort of medicine or therapeutic supervision. If all else fails look for guidance from an affirmed naturopath or doctor. As usual, when starting new herbs or characteristic drugs like Cannabidiol, influence sure to start moderate to fathom how your body reacts and create to higher doses after some time.

Proven Health Benefits of CBD Oil

California was the absolute first state to approve medicinal cannabis in 1996. From that point forward, 27 additional states and Washington, D.C., have really authorized its restorative use.

What's more, after the November 2016 decision, the Golden State went into the 25% of the nation that likewise approaches lawful relaxation pot.

This "green dash for unheard of wealth" is among the best financial patterns today. What's more, it's just a question of time before cannabis use is authorized in some sort the nation over.

California without a doubt started a development on the restorative cannabis front. One where doctors could exhort it as a treatment for seizures, malignant growth, joint pain, ceaseless inconvenience, HIV/AIDS, epilepsy, numerous sclerosis, headaches, resting scatters, nervousness, PTSD, diminished craving and then some.

Research ponders demonstrate that the medicinal favorable circumstances of cannabis are certain. Which's gratitude to substances inside the plant called cannabinoids.

There are in excess of 60 sorts of cannabinoids in maryjane. THC is the most-discussed, as this is the one that offers the hallucinogenic outcomes.

Be that as it may, on the off chance that you don't approach cannabis ... or then again wish to keep away from any of its possibly cerebrum modifying impacts

Give me a chance to introduce you to a different - and legitimate - compound.

It's called cannabidiol, or CBD for short.

CBD is the huge non-psychoactive component of Cannabis sativa. (The clinical term for a sort of cannabis.).

As per a 2013 research examine distributed in the British Journal of Clinical Pharmacology, CBD works as an:.

- Calming.

- Anticonvulsant (or, hostile to seizure agent).

- Cancer prevention agent.

- Antiemetic (agent versus queasiness, development affliction and hurling). Anxiolytic (tension reducer), and.

- Antipsychotic specialist.

just to give some examples...

What's more, CBD oil is totally legitimate because of the way that it very well may be drawn out from hemp, a nearby cousin of cannabis.

Presently, hemp isn't generally legitimate to develop in each U.S. state. Anyway the Food and Drug Administration records CBD oil as a "dietary enhancement." That shows you can get it on the web and have it given to any state.

Amazing Anti-Inflammatory.

I've created to you in many cases about the threats of agony relievers and non-steroidal enemy of inflammatories like Tylenol and Advil.

Standard medications like these can accompany serious physical reactions like ulcers, liver harm and inner dying.

Also, sedative based painkillers like Vicodin and hydrocodone are huge elements to the considerably more-perilous compulsion scourge our nation manages.

Industrious swelling has been connected to disease like malignant growth, heart issue, diabetes, rheumatoid joint pain, neurodegenerative scatters like Alzheimer's, and bunches of others.

In case you're hunting down an option in contrast to the hazardous pharmaceuticals used to treat these kind of conditions, look close to CBD oil.

Studies have really indicated CBD significantly smothers perpetual incendiary and neuropathic inconvenience. What's more, it does as such without activating pain relieving (or, painkiller) resilience.

To puts it basically ...

Not at all like sedative agony relievers- - which just cover torment and quickly develop a resilience in the body- - CBD is an effective mitigating that does not lose its proficiency with time.

Stress and uneasiness Relief.

Another plague by and by destroying the U.S. is our reliance on hurtful pressure and nervousness prescriptions like Xanax, Valium and Ativan.

These are transient arrangements that bring a high danger of enslavement. However, it would appear that some therapeutic experts hand them out like Halloween treat.

CBD oil is a characteristic elective that can be similarly as dependable, without the negative antagonistic impacts.

CBD oil has really been uncovered to bring down pressure and nervousness in customers with social uneasiness condition. Analysts prescribe that it might in like manner work for fit of anxiety, over the top habitual condition, social tension issue and injury.

A 2011 research examine looked at the effects of a reenactment open talking test. Scientists checked solid control customers, and treatment-local customers with social pressure and tension condition.

An in general of 24 never-treated customers with social pressure and uneasiness condition were given either CBD or a fake treatment 1.5 hours before the test.

Researchers found that pre-treatment with CBD fundamentally decreased pressure and uneasiness, psychological incapacity and distress in their discourse productivity.

The fake treatment bunch displayed higher pressure and tension, intellectual weakness and uneasiness.

Diabetes Prevention.

Practically HALF of the U.S populace either has diabetes or uncovers pre-diabetes signs.

This dangerous ailment represents its own everyday medical issues. Anyway it in like manner puts you at a lot more serious hazard for coronary illness, kidney disappointment, nerve harm, and various different clutters.

Studies have discovered that CBD treatment extensively brings down the peril of diabetes in mice. The event dropped from 86% in non-offered mice 30% in CBD-treated mice.

Which means, CBD impactsly affects your glucose and can lessen your danger of diabetes.

Squeamishness.

CBD is a powerful squeamishness and hurling reducer, similarly as cannabis has really been advanced for a considerable length of time.

A 2012 research consider discharged in the British Journal of Pharmacology found that CBD points of interest included enemy of sickness and antiemetic impacts (trust development disease, and chemotherapy reactions) when it was directed.

Next time you're feeling somewhat woozy, don't go after the TUMS or Pepto. Consider this regular substitute rather.

Seizure Treatment.

Cannabis has uncovered on numerous occasions its capacity to manage seizures where different sorts of present day drug have really fizzled.

These exceptional impacts have really been a reviving weep for restorative cannabis supporters. This is among the main powers behind its broad (and endeavor I state "developing") legitimization.

Presently, science is uncovering CBD can give a similar sort of treatment.

For example, a 2014 Stanford University study uncovered great outcomes for the utilization of cannabidiols to treat kids with epilepsy.

A critical note: The normal number of against epileptic medications endeavored before utilizing CBD was 12.

Sixteen of the 19 mothers and fathers (84%) revealed a decrease in their tyke's seizure recurrence while taking CBD cannabis. Of these:.

Two (11%) announced total seizure adaptability.

8 (42%) announced a more noteworthy than 80% decrease in seizure recurrence.

Six (32%) detailed a 25%- - 60% seizure decline.

Other advantageous effects included expanded readiness, much better state of mind and improved rest; while negative impacts included drowsiness and weariness.

Several Other Potential Benefits

CBD has been studied for its role in treating a number of health issues other than those outlined above.

Though more studies are needed, CBD is thought to provide the following health benefits:

• Antipsychotic effects: Studies suggest that CBD may help people with schizophrenia and other mental disorders by reducing psychotic symptoms .

• Substance abuse treatment: CBD has been shown to modify circuits in the brain related to drug addiction. In rats, CBD has been shown to reduce morphine dependence and heroin-seeking behavior .

• Anti-tumor effects: In test-tube and animal studies, CBD has demonstrated anti-tumor effects. In animals, it has been shown to prevent the spread of breast, prostate, brain, colon and lung cancer.

• Diabetes prevention: In diabetic mice, treatment with CBD reduced the incidence of diabetes by 56% and significantly reduced inflammation .

GOOD NEWS

Hemp Cannabidiol (CBD) products have been approved by the government of Brazil as a treatment for cancer. High grade CBD has also been approved by Brazil as a prescription medication for the treatment of epilepsy, Parkinson's disease, and other types of serious chronic pain. This move puts Brazil far ahead of the United States in the realm of compassionate, safe, affordable medicine that can treat serious medical conditions such as cancer.

This is just the beginning to your education. I sincerely hope you will continue to search for and find a wide range of useful holistic remedies to be happy and healthy your entire life.

Made in United States
Orlando, FL
27 April 2024

46253546R00046